Down Syndrome: Raising a Child Like Kimmy

Judith E. Mathewson

Strategic Book Publishing
New York, New York

Copyright © 2009

All rights reserved – Judith Mathewson

No part of this book may be reproduced or transmitted in any form or by any means, graphic, electronic, or mechanical, including photocopying, recording, taping, or by any information storage retrieval system, without the permission, in writing, from the publisher.

Strategic Book Publishing
An imprint of Writers Literary & Publishing Services, Inc.
845 Third Avenue, 6th Floor – 6016
New York, NY 10022

http://www.strategicbookpublishing.com

ISBN: 978-1-60860-193-6

Printed in the United States of America

Dedication

This book is dedicated to all the parents of special needs children. As you read this book, I pray that you will gain knowledge, encouragement, and hope. God has directed these writings, and my hope is that Kimmy's story will bless all the people who read this book.

I want to thank all my friends and family for their support and love throughout our lives. They have encouraged me to share this true story of Kimmy and the path that God has given her. With God's blessings, she has touched the lives of all those individuals who have had the courage to get to know her.

Contents

Chapter 1: The Birth of an Angel 1

Chapter 2: Difficult Months Ahead 9

Chapter 3: Survival 21

Chapter 4: The Progressive Years 37

Chapter 5: Personality Plus 49

Chapter 6: Southern Living 55

Chapter 7: Expectations—Have None! 63

Appendix A: Emergency Information Record and
   Authorization for Emergency Treatment 71

Appendix B: Personal Care Instructions. 73

Chapter 1

The Birth of an Angel

In November 1966, Kimberly Anne was conceived. At the tender age of twenty-one, my life was suddenly flowing with excitement, uncertainty, and love as she grew inside the comfort and protection of my womb.

I had no conception of what it meant to have an O negative blood type. Since the doctor did not seem alarmed, it must not be anything to be concerned about. Red flags should have gone off in my head alerting me that type O negative blood was not good for my unborn baby and that this needed to be looked into. This Rh factor and the fact that my husband had the blood type of B positive was a major issue for the unborn baby. That the doctor should have done more tests, blood work, and that he should have made the recommendation of "amniocentesis" tests. But, this had never occurred to me.

Kimmy was born in July 1967, two days after my birthday, which, in my mind, made her an extra special gift from God. With a birth weight of four pounds, fourteen ounces, she was placed into an incubator until her weight had stabilized near five pounds. Once Kimmy reached that goal, the nurses let me hold my daughter. I called her "my little monkey" since she had olive colored skin like my dad and me. She had brown hair and slightly slanted, pretty brown eyes—again so much like my eyes. I believed my daughter to be absolutely perfect. The nurses explained that Kimmy did not have the sucking power to nurse from my breast because she was four weeks premature. However, she never drank milk from a bottle for me either. I thought this strange, but the nurses assured me that they had just given her a bottle, so she most likely was not hungry. Nodding, I would turn my attention back to Kimmy, "My Little Angel."

Ten days after her birth, Kimmy's weight reached four pounds, fifteen ounces. With this milestone, the nurses announced that once the doctor came in and signed the release papers, we could go home. What an exciting moment for us! Those ten days seemed like months, and I was anxious to go home with my perfect baby girl.

While I was packing and getting ready for our trip home, the pediatrician made his only visit during my ten-day stay at the hospital. When he came in, he asked me two questions. First, "Do you love your baby?" I thought this was an odd, but an easy to answer, question. Then he asked, "What is your home phone number?" Again, an easy answer. Without another word, he turned and left. I resumed packing and laying out the clothes and blanket for Kimmy's trip home. I again thought how strange for the doctor to ask if I loved my baby. And why ask for my phone number? Wouldn't my hospital file have our home phone number? I brushed the thought aside. We were going home, which was all that mattered.

Without my knowledge, the pediatrician had called my husband to tell him that he could pick up his wife and Down syndrome daughter. There was no explanation, no advice, no guidance, no caring—just those harsh, cold, straightforward words!

After my husband picked us up, we had one stop to make. We needed to purchase baby bottles, a sterilizer, and other necessities needed for bottle feeding since breast nursing was not a choice. After arriving home, I laid Kimmy down in her pretty, ruffled covered crib to sleep. My husband then asked me to sit down on the couch because he wanted to tell me something. Immediately, my thoughts were that he was going to tell me that he loved me and missed me. But, he only spoke to me about Kimmy being a Down syndrome baby. He was not sure what degree of mongolism she had, he only knew that the doctor told him his wife and Down syndrome child were ready to go home.

Tears filled my eyes as I said, "She'll never grow into childhood, never go on a date, never go to a prom, and never get married and have children of her own. She would never experience what this life has to offer her."

But I was wrong! She has a peace, joy, love, and trust that others will never be able to experience. She also possesses an incredible amount of unconditional love.

After various tests and x-rays, the doctors confirmed that Kimmy had Down syndrome. The doctors also suggested that I would have a one in a million chance of having a normal child. Although these odds were extremely high, the desire for another child was strong. A second child would be loved whether disabled or normal. Seven months after the birth of

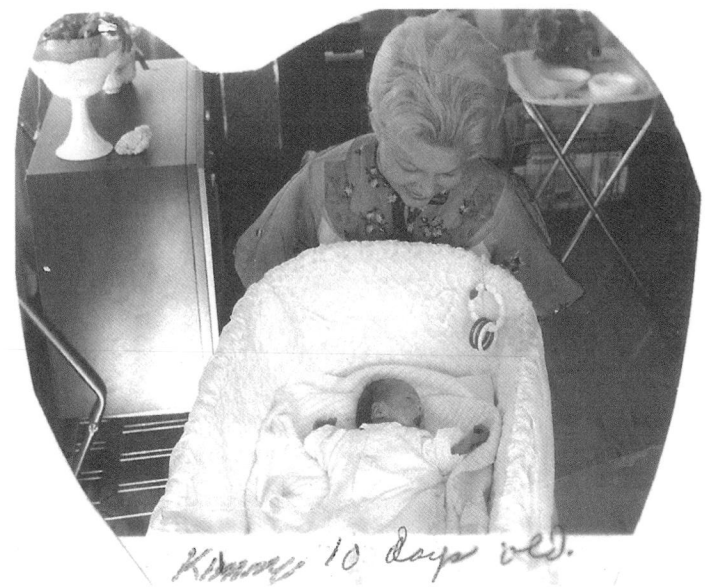

Kimmy, 10 days old, with Grandma Mathewson

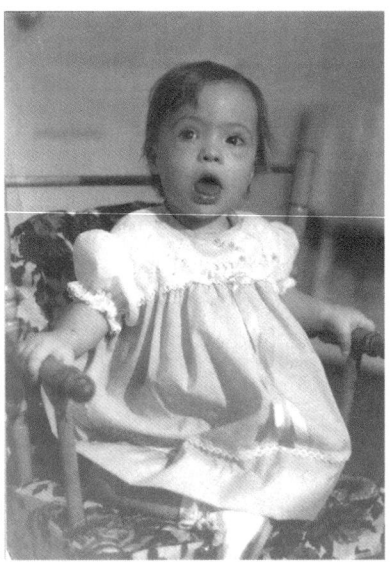

Kimmy, 2 years old

Kimmy, our second child, Suzanne Eileen was conceived. During this pregnancy, the baby had undergone four amniocentesis tests. During this process, a small amount of amniotic fluid was removed from the sac surrounding the fetus. This helped the doctors keep track of her physical development. Along with keeping an eye on those issues, the doctors watched the baby's blood type and knew that "premature labor" was going to cause a short-term pregnancy. This kept the doctors extremely busy.

An additional complication occurred when my water broke six weeks prior to our second child's anticipated birth date, which would have been around Christmas. When my water broke, this caused an endangerment to her life; therefore, the doctors quickly made the decision to induce labor. Suzanne was born in November 1968, weighing in at a low four pounds, eleven ounces. As a premature baby, she was placed in an incubator and had to remain in the hospital for two weeks after I was released. I was faced with not being able to take Suzanne home immediately, returning to an abusive husband, and experiencing hormonal changes. But, I also faced postpartum depression. When Suzanne was able to come home, she did not receive the full attention that a baby needs and requires. Kimberly, too, required so much of my attention, that I was overwhelmed.

But God was merciful. My husband showed affection and attention to Suzanne that he did not have for me or Kimmy. It was not until she was six years old and learned right from wrong that she became fearful and scared. Raising two children would keep any mother busy and stretched to her limits. If one of the children is disabled, the pressures and fatigue escalate.

In March 1969, four months after the birth of Suzanne, I realized I was pregnant with a third baby. This was totally unexpected, but it took away some of the distractions of caring for two children and dealing with an abusive situation. People would ask me about the marks on my body, but I would just state that I had fallen down or walked into a door. I knew if I told them the truth and he found out I would get abused even worse. He'd tell me I liked it, or that if I would just do what I was told he wouldn't need to hit me. So for the sake of the babies I continually tried to make him as pleased with me as possible.

When I was four weeks pregnant with my third child, the doctors at a university hospital thought it best to abort the baby. The eleven doctors had discussed my case history and believed that the baby would likely be born physically or mentally disabled.

They told me that this baby had only a one in a million chance of being born normal. They explained that my first child, Kimberly, was born with Down syndrome when I was only twenty-two. They further explained that my O-negative blood and past "premature labor" births would shorten the normal nine-month pregnancy. Their calculations showed that my pregnancy term would be seven-and-a-half to eight months and promised little chance of survival.

The doctors stated that my second daughter, Suzanne, had been fortunate to have been born normal. However, in their professional opinion, these tests indicated that my third baby would not be so fortunate. The doctors scheduled the abortion to be done the next week while the pregnancy was still in its early stages.

As I drove home, I contemplated their prognosis. Thoughts about this little unborn life within me kept going through my mind. Should this abortion happen? All signs concurred, but my heart felt otherwise.

I thank God that He intervened in my thoughts during the week prior to the scheduled abortion. When I returned to the hospital to meet with the doctors, I had the strength to state that there would be no abortion. If this child was born disabled or with Down syndrome, I would take care of this baby with the love and care that I was giving both Kimmy and Suzanne. I could not give up on this unborn child. This baby deserved to be loved and cared for.

During the seven months of pregnancy the usual amniocentesis tests and lab blood work was done. But with this pregnancy the doctors were very concerned with the babies blood. Everything was happening at one time, the baby wanted out, her blood was bad, she needed a blood transfusion immediately and the pregnancy was only at the 7th month term. The doctors shifted into high gear deciding on what options they had to choose to perform the needed blood transfusion and yet still have a safe baby delivery.

My doctors stated that if she was going to live, she needed to build up her strength. There were two options. My baby could "fight" her way out, which meant inducing labor. Or the doctors could attempt the blood transfusion while she was still within my womb. However, if that was not successful, it could also cause her death.

The decision was easy. Inducing labor gave her the greatest chance of survival and provided the increased need of strength to bring her into this world. In September 1969, two months short of a full term, labor was induced. After the birth, the doctors would begin the necessary blood transfusions. Tamara Jeanne was born in September 1969, weighing in at five pounds. Her blood type was a mixture of B positive and O negative. Doctors state that a combination both blood types present in the child would be of danger to her life, causing "yellow jaundice," would be one of the effects. Therefore, it was absolutely necessary to continue with as many blood transfusions as necessary to get her out of this danger zone.

Things never go quite as straightforward as planned, one transfusion turned into two. And with each transfusion, the doctors asked if they could baptize her. Those words frightened me. The second transfusion turned into a third transfusion, and once more I was asked if they could baptize her again. Tears welled up in my eyes as I nodded yes. She was barely holding on, but I knew God continued to watch over her.

As the doctors and nurses prepared her for the third transfusion, she started to come out of the danger zone. That meant that the third blood transfusion was not needed. Seven days later, I left the hospital with my blonde, brown-eyed, normal baby girl who now weighed in at five pounds and six ounces. And so, she became another miracle child.

Chapter 2

Difficult Months Ahead

The early weeks of caring for Kimmy were pure torture for me as a first-time mother. No one gave me information on her exact health condition, I was only informed that she was a Down syndrome baby. And, no nurse or doctor offered to instruct me on how to care for her. No one explained what health signs should alert me to take her to an emergency room for treatment or observation.

Caring for a first child is difficult enough as you attempt to do everything just right. Caring for a disabled child is even more difficult. Her life depended on my vigilance. Her daily health condition could and did change drastically. As I watched and waited for any changes that may occur, I never knew if she would make it through the rough days. As with many first-time mothers, much of what I learned was by trial and error. My main goal was to keep her alive and nourished. I needed to keep her limp, lifeless, frail arms and legs moving by bending them back and forth. I lifted her wobbly little head to strengthen her neck muscles. I found this to be the most difficult since her head wobbled from side to side and back and forth. By placing my fingertips behind her head and at the base of her neck, I gently used a forward and backward motion trying to strengthen the muscles that lacked any control. This was all that could be done for that area of the body, and this became our daily routine.

Crying is a way for babies to exercise their lungs, but Kimmy rarely cried. Her breathing was so shallow that I would place her by the side of my bed at night. Periodically, I would wake up to see if her little chest was moving up and down and to check her heartbeat. This pattern of shallow breathing caused her doctors to be even more thorough during her regular six-month checkups. Her life depended on the strength of her lungs and heart to keep her body running as efficiently as possible.

At the age of six months, Kimmy was still quite small and weighed just ten pounds, ten ounces. Her arms and legs were only the size of my baby finger. But her stomach protruded from fluid retention, so much so, that she looked as though she was seven months pregnant. On her first birthday, she weighted fourteen pounds. Her arms and legs now were the size of my thumb, but the stomach protruded less because of the water pills the doctors had prescribed for her.

Bottle feeding remained a challenge since she had no sucking power. I developed a system to feed her the milk that was so vital to keeping her alive. By slightly enlarging the hole of the bottle's nipple and pinching the sides of it, I could get a few drops of milk onto her thick tongue. All Down syndrome babies have enlarged tongues. It is one of their traits. The tongue protrudes out of the mouth due to the fact that it is larger than the mouth. With Kimmy, I thought it was cute, so I would smile at her and tap my finger on the tip of her tongue causing her to laugh and instinctively pull the tongue back into her mouth. Her laughing at this became a game and over the years it would benefit her because she learned to hold her tongue in her mouth. To help her drink from her bottle, I would rub my finger up and down her throat so she would automatically swallow. It took approximately one hour for her to drink a couple ounces of milk. This procedure was repeated every three hours, twenty-four hours a day. I would wake automatically during the night, pick her up, and feed and rock her. Then knowing there was nothing else that could be done, I'd cry. I cried for her, for her life, and my ability to care for her. My thoughts centered on whether I would or could keep her alive.

After three weeks, I made a call to my pediatrician's office and asked to speak to him. It was only a week until Kimmy's four-week checkup, but I needed his advice before the appointment date since I felt Kimmy's life depended on it. When he answered the phone, I explained who I was and that I needed his input on how to care for Kimmy. I needed to know if what I was doing was okay in his opinion. He flatly answered, "You should put her into an institution. That is my recommendation. Now don't call me again!" Just as abruptly, he hung up on me.

After crying hysterically, I called my mom, who suggested finding another pediatrician. My next phone call was to a friend, who was a nurse and lived nearby. I am sure that I sounded like a babbling idiot trying to explain the problem to her through my hysteria. She gave me the name of a doctor. She was confident that this doctor would take good care of

Kimmy, run tests, and help me learn how to meet Kimmy's needs.

After explaining the situation and my desperate plea for help, Doctor Mary Kenly (not her real name), set up an appointment to see Kimmy the following day. She agreed with the diagnosis that Kimmy was a Down syndrome baby. She showed me the palm of Kimmy's little hand with the middle line that reached from one side to the opposite side of the palm. Everyone has two lines on the palm, but a child with Down syndrome will always have one line that will go completely across the palm, this is just one of many indicators of a Down syndrome child. She proceeded to show me the tiny little ear traits, the slight slant of the eyes, and the round facial features that are characteristic with Down syndrome.

Doctor Mary Kenly was an answer to my prayers, she was one of God's angels sent from heaven. With patience, kindness, knowledge, and caring she took my daughter under her gentle wings for the first three years of Kimmy's life.

But, she also stated that to know the full extent of Kimmy's health condition tests would need to be performed at a hospital. When we arrived, the nurses, lab technicians, and doctors were all very kind and professional. They carefully explained the tests, x- rays, and blood work as we went along.

Kimmy was pricked, probed, turned, and put into plastic tubes while I held her up by her tiny hands and arms as an x-ray machine encircled her small frail body like a capsule. She was frightened so I spoke to her calmly and in a loving voice. She relaxed somewhat and her eyes searched my face for signs of concern. Is it possible that she sensed my inner fears and terrors?

These tests not only confirmed Down syndrome, but they also revealed two holes on the same side of her heart (upper and lower chambers). This meant that her heart was working overtime pumping blood forcefully past these holes into the arteries. Left untreated, this would cause a buildup of scar tissue over the years in her arteries. In turn, this would reduce the diameter of her arteries and weaken the heart. In 1967, heart operations were not performed as easily or as frequently as they are now. We lived one day at a time not knowing if there would be a next day for Kimmy. Love was all I could give her. No doctor could predict her life span. As she grew, we became best buds, laughing, hugging, and playing little games. She has always been my "little angel." She was my blessing from God and the best gift He could ever have given me. So we lived the first ten years of her life rushing to the doctor's office or going directly to hospital emergency rooms every few months. I would let the hospital know when we were on our way, and they would have a room set up for her according to the doctor's orders. At various times, Kimmy was diagnosed with pneumonia, bronchitis, or dehydration. Sometimes, her diagnosis used medical terms that were foreign to me. Other times, she would have a combination of illnesses. Since her resistance level was low, she was highly susceptible to viruses and illnesses. This required that she be quarantined in a separate room from other children so not to complicate her own condition.

Often I heard the words, "Now you know, Mrs. Mathewson, there is little chance she will live through this sickness. Her system is just not capable of handling more illnesses, so all we can do is keep her on intravenous feeding, medication, and make her comfortable. As you are aware, she lives on a moment-by-moment basis. You must prepare for the worst and hope for the best. She might be able to fight through this sickness, but we have to prepare you for the inevitable." My heart would sink every time I heard those words. I never got used to them. But Kimmy had a drive to live, and my drive for her survival was as strong as hers.

The doctors had stated that Kimmy's projected physical outlook did not look good. There were no guarantees that she would have the ability or strength to walk or even talk. She defied that prognosis too. She was using the baby walker at two; by three and a half, she had worn out four baby walkers. Kimmy could not crawl like a normal child does. To get around on the floor, she would grab the shag carpeting and then pull herself forward. Her brain did not make the connection to the legs to tell them to move. Plus, she had no strength in those little legs. When Kimmy was a baby, I added routine leg work into her daily exercise program. She would pull herself up to try to stand on those weak legs then she would attempt to push them against my belly to a standing position. Kimmy did not stand on her own until she was three years old. She did not have the leg strength to hold her body up. When she was a baby, I would encourage her to strengthen her legs by holding her around her chest and helping her lift herself up to a standing position. These exercises strengthened the leg muscles. Her arms were strengthened by just pumping them at the elbow and rotating her little shoulder sockets around in a circle.

Kimmy's baby sister, Suzy, was six months old and crawling everywhere. Suzy and I would get down on all fours to show Kimmy the motions of how to crawl. But, she would just smile with an ear-to-ear grin, lay down on the floor, and pull herself across the floor.

How she made it from a flat position to a sitting position amazed everyone. Lying on her stomach, she brought her legs straight out and then swung them flat on the floor to stretch out beside her. It looked as though her legs were attached to the sides of her body, not her hip sockets. She would proceed to put her hands in front of her and push herself up, legs still out to her side. The last part of the process was to swing her legs straight out in front of her and finish by bending her knees to balance into a sitting position. Ouch! We would all grin and shake our heads in amazement at her determination and flexibility. Those exercises helped her. But she really gained strength when she could grab the floor with her tippy toes when she was in her baby walker. This was monumental progress—and she knew it. Kimmy would look at me and smile with a self-satisfied ear-to-ear grin that any mother would treasure. Little accomplishments like this were major steps in her life. And those accomplishments encouraged her to keep going.

When she was about two years old, I suddenly awoke from an afternoon nap on the couch. I had been dreaming and was now sobbing. Kimmy had appeared in my dreams in little white tights, ruffled lace panties, tiny white baby shoes, and a white dress embroidered in green and red. In my dream, she was running to me from across the room. At that time, it was pure agony to have a dream like that.

Kimmy did take her first precious baby steps when she was four years old. It wasn't until after those first steps that I realized that God had given me that dream to show me that she would walk. And that dream remains as a reminder that God does answer our prayers as well as our desires and hopes. He gives us visions in dreams as though He is speaking directly to us. We just need to be still and quiet and know to listen.

If Kimmy hadn't walked, if it was not in God's plan, I would have accepted that. For He will never give us more than we are able to handle—even when we think we cannot handle any more.

There were times when Kimmy was limp as a rag and white as a sheet. At these times, she was unresponsive to anything around her and was content to just lay there unmoving. When Kimmy was four, she went into a coma. I thought she was sleeping on the couch, as she sometimes liked to do just to be around me, but when the nap was half an hour longer than usual, I went to check on her. That is when I found I could not get her to wake up and rushed her to the hospital. The doctor who had been so compassionate and caring gently told me that Kimmy would not live through this episode. As always, I slept by Kimmy's side. Sometimes I slept in a chair or would spread out under her crib, but I never left her alone. I would reach inside the oxygen tent that surrounded her crib, and talk to her and pat her back. I never knew if she could hear me. But I prayed that somehow she could and would feel my love.

Kimmy did survive this four-day coma. When she could breathe on her own, relief consumed me. I climbed up into her hospital crib, and wrapped my arms around her and fell fast asleep. Sitting or laying on a patient's bed (a crib in our case) was clearly frowned on. A nurse later told me that when she walked by and saw me sleeping and Kimmy patting my back, she couldn't bring herself to separate us. I still get chills when I recall the nurse telling me how Kimmy patted my back, she said it was like Kimmy was reassuring and comforting me. It was her way of letting me know, "It's all right now Mommy, you can rest. I'm here by your side."

During those four days in the hospital, I talked to God a lot. He continually reminded me that He let Kimmy live and that He had heard my prayers. He also wanted me to write a book about her so others would have an understanding about Down syndrome children. He wanted others to know the joys and the sorrows that come from raising and loving a child like Kimmy—my Down syndrome child and the love of my life. He wanted her story to be told so that others could have help and hope. He wanted others to know there is a God and He is watching over us. He hears our cries and will answer us. But, He may not always answer in the way we expect to be answered. But the answer always benefits the kingdom of God. He will pour out His love and comfort upon us so we can make it through any situation that may arise.

I know this to be true because my first marriage of ten years and two months was an abusive marriage. I knew of no help for my situation at that time. I remember those times with a great deal of sadness as I was pregnant the first 3 years of our marriage.

As often is the case with the abuser, my husband blamed me for his behavior. Any psychologist or shelter or police officer will concur that the attacker blames the victim. And the one who is being abused is willing to change anything that may end the abuse. So the victims shoulder the blame. The victims convince themselves that if they could change, the abuser would show love and the abuse would end.

But that never happened. I had three children in twenty-six months. Our first child, Kimmy, was born with Down syndrome, the second two were healthy.

God gave me these three children. He knew that for us to survive, love would need to flow between us. That no matter what might happen, we would have each other. And we did. My three beautiful daughters and I played, laughed, cooked, danced, and grew up together. When they were old enough to be frightened for me, they would scream and cry. I knew I had to protect them and myself. In 1977, I ended the marriage. Raising children while living in an abusive marriage is not healthy for anyone. If you are in a situation of abuse to yourself or your children, I pray that you will talk to your pastor, a counselor, a police officer, or seek out a shelter for abused women. Don't allow yourself or your children to be victimized. The problem is not yours—it is the abuser's.

Out of a disastrous marriage, I finally began to raise my girls while living a peaceful, normal life. And raise them I did! However, if it had not been for Suzanne and Tammy helping me with Kimmy, I don't know how I could have done it—but God knew. He blessed me with Suzanne and Tammy as much as He had blessed me with Kimmy.

As the years have passed, Suzanne and Tamara have continued to be there for Kimmy and me. Distance has not been a factor; only how fast they can get to me and Kimmy is the factor. And this will remain till God takes us home and cares for us with His loving hands.

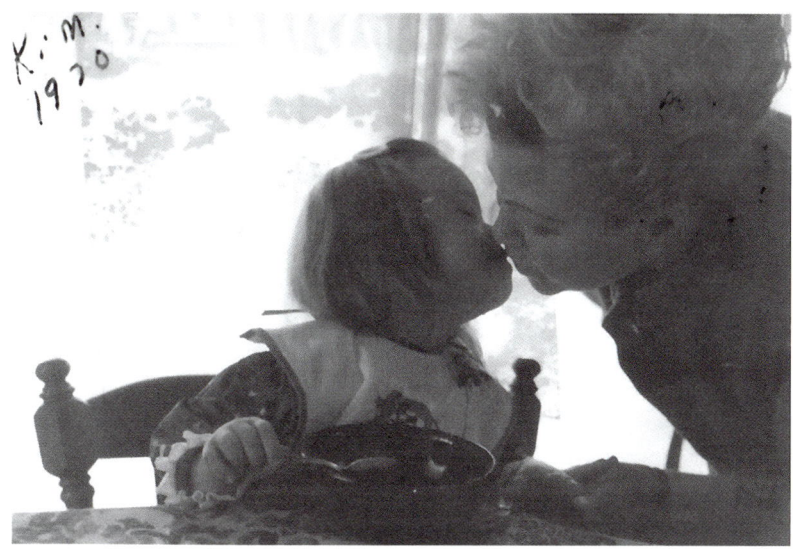

Kimmy, 3 years old, smooching Grandma Mathewson

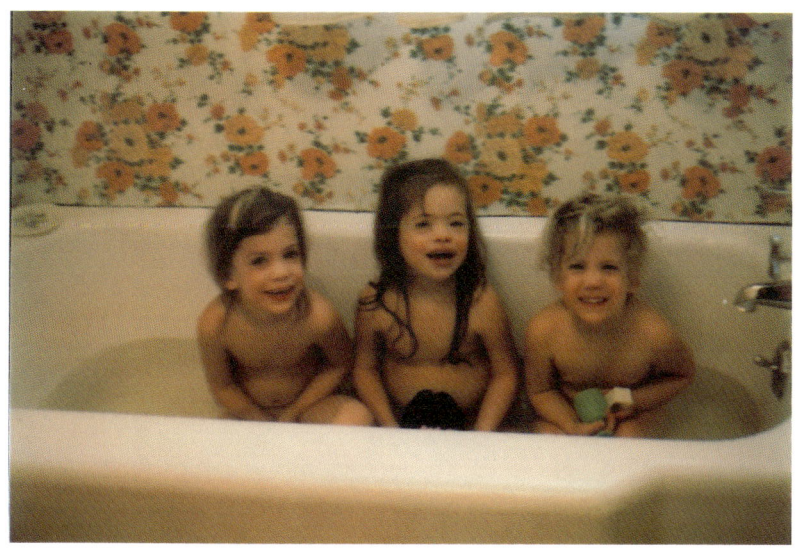

Kimmy, 4 years old, with sisters Suzy and Tammy

Chapter 3

Survival

Kimmy's first ten years of life can be summed up in one word, survival. Kimmy fought for her life those first ten years. She also defied what the doctors had predicted for her life expectancy. Kimmy's desire to live and the love she felt from me, my mother, and others has kept her just as precious and beautiful as she was when she came into this world forty-one years ago.

She had an extraordinary will to live and to be with those who loved her. Naturally, she and I had a strong attachment to one another. But she also had a strong attachment to my mother, her grandma.

My mother always had that intuition (or feeling some would say) when she knew something was wrong with Kimmy. A phone call would confirm her feelings. My parents would close up their business and drive the four to six hours (depending on where we lived at the time) to stay with us until those danger days passed and Kimmy could return home for the remainder of her recovery period.

My mother was great that way. She was always there to give me encouragement and lavish her love and care upon her granddaughter. In 2005, my mother took care of Kimmy for four days at my home so I could attend a wedding in Florida. While I was away, the car she was driving was hit by a pickup truck that was going too fast in a residential area. She died four days later in the trauma center at a university hospital in Michigan.

I not only lost my mother, but Kimmy lost someone who loved her unconditionally. My mother possessed a strong commitment to love and care for Kimmy. She easily gave up part of her personal life to be there for her granddaughter. I have always wanted to be like my mom and have her strength, love of God, caring, and the sacrificial giving of self to family and friends. I hope she is looking down from heaven even now, smiling upon me and Kimmy knowing how much she is loved and missed by us. She has had a tremendous impact on our lives.

It was often tough jostling two healthy babies to friends' houses while rushing Kimmy to hospitals and emergency rooms. However, I believe that it turned my daughters into the strong and caring individuals they are to this day.

My husband never took care of the children. When I needed to go grocery shopping, run errands, or do other wifely and motherly duties, I would take all three babies with me. Until Kimmy was four and Tammy was two, I'd carry both of them in my arms and Suzy would hang onto my miniskirt. Looking back on it makes me smile for we must have made quite a scene to the surrounding onlookers. There were times, when the children were younger, that people would ask if I had triplets.

That's truly what it looked like and sometimes I felt that way, too. But, this was our way of life. This was how we made it through those years. We took care of each other, laughing and loving as much as we could under our circumstances.

When my husband would go out in the evening to a bar, he would leave me home, but not before saying, "You wanted the kids, so you take care of them! And besides it would cost twice as much if I took you along, even if our neighbor did agree to watch them." So it was either the bar or gambling or hunting with his buddies that kept him off on his own. I learned to accept the situation for the well being of the babies and myself.

For Kimmy, hospitals, emergency rooms, doctors, nurses, needles, feeding tubes, and having her wrists and ankles tied down became a normal part of her life. Almost like clockwork, she'd be back in the hospital every four months with bronchitis, pneumonia, dehydration, or a virus that attacked her compromised health and her fragile immune system. Vomiting was a regular occurrence. When she would begin to gag, Suzy and Tammy would run toward the bathroom for towels to spread lengthwise in front of Kimmy. I held one up in front under her chin to catch the spew of vomit. It was inconceivable how such a small child could project vomit up to six feet with such force. If the dehydration was so severe that I could not alter it by giving her lots of fluids, I had to take her to the hospital were they would start her on IVs. There were times when hospitalization was not necessary and watching her for signs of urgency was enough. But the decision whether or not to go to the hospital was a fine line in the decision-making process. Her health, abilities, and the severity of the situation all depended on what decision I would make for the situation at hand. Once again, I would ask God's guidance and pray that Kimmy would make it through, yet again, another illness.

In the winter months, Kimmy's immune system was more susceptible to viruses and germs, which meant that going outside to play with her sisters was out of the question. So Kimmy would sit at the kitchen table laughing and screeching with glee when Suzy or Tammy would throw snowballs, not only at each other, but tossed a few at the window where Kimmy was watching.

Although she had problems with her health and the cold weather, Kimmy was an easy child to care for. She had a happy and mild disposition, rarely cried, and loved life and the people who were in her life. Kimmy loved everyone and those who took the time to know Kimmy, loved her in return.

There were times when people did not know how to relate to her or pulled away because of her disability, but Kimmy's love would remain steadfast and giving. Sometimes I wished I had her ability to accept people and situations the way that she did in her everyday life! What a gift from God to love unconditionally! I can't help but think that if everyone were blessed with that ability, I am sure we would look, act, and feel differently than we do right now.

Though people loved her, she had only her sisters and me to play with her. However, when she was seven years old, she was able to attend a Pied Piper school for disabled or special needs children. She would get on the little yellow ("lellow" is how she pronounces that color) bus and go to a world only she, the teachers, and other students understood. It takes very dedicated individuals to give of themselves to work with and teach children who have special needs. I appreciate and praise them for giving of themselves selflessly and for their ability to work with and relate to those who are physically or mentally challenged.

Kimmy attended the Pied Piper School from the time she was seven until she was eighteen. At that time, her lung capacity to breathe worsened. While a healthy person can breathe at an oxygen level of 96, Kimmy was capable of breathing only at a much lower level of 76. The doctor wrote up the prescription for an oxygen medical equipment company to supply her with the necessary oxygen concentrator for home use and tanks of oxygen for use outside the home such as shopping, doctor appointments, family visits, etc. As her oxygen level decreased in her body, she began to be governed by her natural secondary activity level. This meant that she was less active. She slept longer at night, took three-hour naps, and was involved in sedentary activities such as polishing clam shells till they were shiny and paper thin. I still have those clam shells boxed up and kept in a special place. I also put together a very special scrapbook of the various things she made or wrote during the day that kept her occupied and mentally challenged. These are the memories that a parent cherishes and holds onto for a lifetime.

Kimmy could no longer be as active as she had been. She no longer rode her bicycle, played basketball, hit a baseball, or was able to swim (which she loved to do so much), or rollerblade. She no longer was able to do many of the home activities that kept her life full. Kimmy's body had become her dictator. She adapted to this secondary activity level as if she had always lived at this level. Despite all the setbacks, her life was full. It is amazing to me how God gives us the ability to adapt to our bodily health needs, as well as to other situations that make up our daily lives.

As Kimmy adjusted positively to her new physical condition, that same positivity spilled over to me. As alarming as her new condition was to me, she was the real trouper (as usual) in making lemonade out of lemons as my mother would say.

Kimmy will always remain at the center of my life. As those of you who have a special needs child know, there is not a second in the day that your child is not on your mind. Like me, you may have put decades of caring, loving, and giving, or you may have had just a few days or months. But, whatever the amount of time you are allotted will be the special time that God has given to you to enjoy and grow together in love. Kimmy has been my true gift from God, but there have been times I have not felt worthy of receiving such a precious gift in my life.

Her sisters have also been a gift. Through all of Kimmy's health scares, learning curves, and daily life experiences, they have been steadfast in their love and caring. Suzy and Tammy have willingly given up part of their life to meet the needs of their older sister.

Like most mothers of children with special needs, we tend to be more protective and hover over them so that they are unable to spread their wings and experience some of the normalcies in life. Balance came through to Kimmy's life with friends and family members who provided other activities and experiences. Most importantly, they took the time to speak, discuss, and talk with Kimmy about her likes and dislikes as if she were as normal as them. They took the time to ask about her day and listen to her response or do those simple things that a parent might not always take the time to do or provide for them during their daily life.

It is incredible how every person has a special gift to impart on another person's life whether it be personal growth, learning, playing, or just plain friendship. What is most amazing is that the more we give the more we receive in return without even knowing that it is happening.

Suzy and Tammy have been able to do this for Kimmy. They bring activities, places, and adventure into Kimmy's life. This is also true for two very special sisters who came into Kimmy's life when she was seventeen. Erin and Jamie lived year-round at a lake where we had just bought an old cottage next to them. They would come over and play board games with Kimmy. Sometimes they invited her to their house to watch videos or take her swimming and play on the large tube in the lake. At the time, it amazed me that God had given Kimmy these two special people into her life. I was thankful for them, but I could never understand why He had not given her other children to play with before this time in her life.

About six years later, Erin went off to college and Jamie was killed in a car accident at the age of seventeen. Everyone was shocked. Jamie was a beautiful, caring, and sensitive child, which made her death even more tragic. God knows why these things happen in life; He has His plan, but sometimes it is difficult to not ask Him, "Why God?" Yet, we must not ask why, but trust in all things that come our way in this life. He has His purpose and we are part of His plan. What makes it difficult is what we do not understand. Then we truly need to trust in Him and lay ourselves, and others that we love, down at His feet.

God heard my prayers asking for Kimmy to have friends in her life and intervened again. When Kimmy was thirty-four years old, God brought five-year-old Ryan and his sister, four-year-old Allison into Kimmy's life. Their parents, Mary Ann and Andrew, were friends of ours and had learned that they could not conceive children. But they were able to adopt two darling children from Russia, Ryan and Allison. At the time of adoption, Ryan was two and his sister Allison was six months old, they both had blue eyes and blonde hair. With the love of their new parents, they adjusted to their new lives in America. As the adult friendships grew, so did the children's friendship with Kimmy. With Ryan, Allison, and their parents, the Fourth of July was a special day. Kimmy was always included and everyone made sure she participated in the fun and the food. All of us enjoyed the boat and pontoon rides to the sand bar. Sometimes, we just cruised around the lake and enjoyed the peace of the setting sun. Taking time out of our life to share and give of ourselves is what life is all about. And, of course, no Fourth of July would be complete without sparklers, bonfires, marshmallows, smiles, and laughter. These are special memories that will be held in our hearts forever.

We remain good friends. Mary Ann and Andrew taught their children the patience and caring that has helped them become the special individuals they are today. They brought these qualities into their relationship with Kimmy, which has helped her to blossom in areas that she might never have had the chance to achieve in her life.

Ryan and Allison spent many hours with Kimmy. They would color, play cards, make crafts, paint, watch TV or videos, play board games, or play with Lady-Di (our little white Maltese). Allison really loved the dog and Lady-Di loved the attention. Ryan and Allison not only played with Kimmy, they made her feel equal, which is an aspect that is so important for other people to understand. They hold a special spot in my heart for the unconditional love they gave to Kimmy.

Regardless of their physical and mental attributes, they have a lot of love to give. All you have to do is reach out to talk to them. Ask them what they like to do, what places they have traveled to, what activities they like, what they like to watch on TV. Ask them about themselves, make them feel important, and show them that you care about them. They have much to give and can make a difference in this world with what they have to offer.

Another special friend is Jena. Even though her children were in high school and college when we first met, Jena, Tom, and their family loved Kimmy and doted on her. Whenever we did things together, they made sure that Kimmy was included and enjoying herself. That always meant so much to me when others loved Kimmy and accepted her for who she is. Jena is a special person. I love her for the individual she has allowed God to form her into spiritually and as a person. Jena has always made it perfectly clear to me that she would care for Kimmy anytime I had to be away whether it was for an hour or several days. She would bring us food when I couldn't get out when Kimmy was so sick that she required my round-the-clock attention.

When Kimmy is sickly she must have someone with her all the time. On days that she is not sick I can leave her at the house for a couple of hours. This is the time I use to run errands. Kimmy has her own cell phone, so if she needs me she only needs to push #1 on her phone and she'll connect to my cell phone; or I call her periodically during running the errands. This gives her comfort as well as myself.

Jena also understood the stress level of my personal life. She was there to help with Kimmy or for me in general. Sometimes, Jena would get pushy with me. She knew that it was hard for me to accept help, as it still is. Jena made me realize that there were times I just had to let others reach out to us. By not doing so, I was keeping others from receiving a blessing from God.

In 1979, I remarried. During our marriage, Russ made Kimmy's life joyful with his gentle teasing. He and Kimmy shared various experiences that she still remembers. Some of those moments were captured in pictures. My hope is that these pictures will touch your heart and perhaps change the way you react to a disabled person.

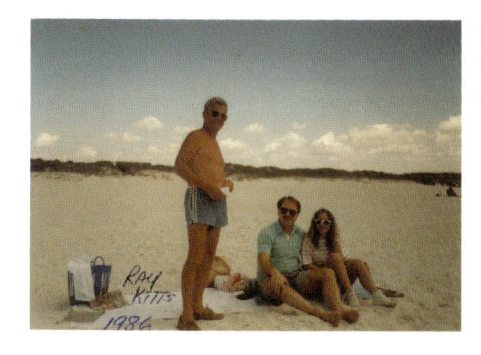

Kimmy, 19 years old, with Ray Kitts and Russ (Dad) at Panama City

1988: family friends Mary Rajasekhar and daughter Rebeca

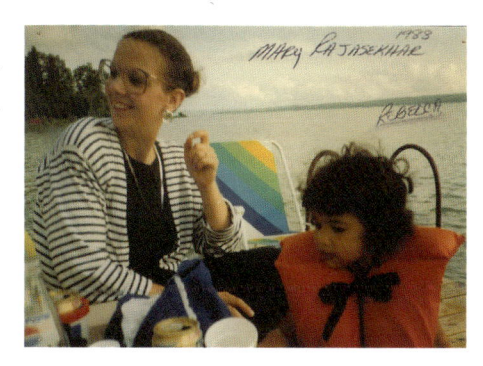

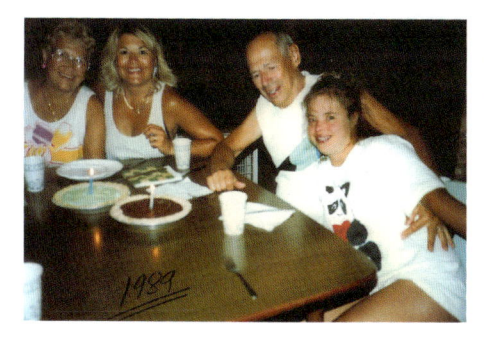

Kimmy, 22 years old, with Grandma, Mom, and Grandpaa

32   *Down Syndrome: Raising a Child Like Kimmy*

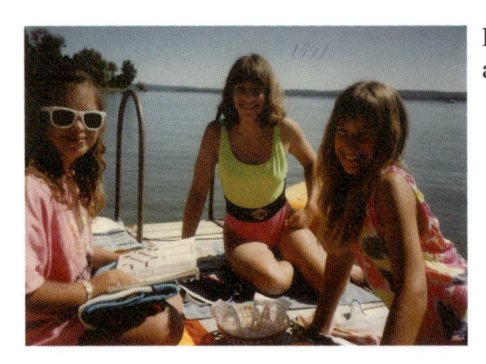

Kimmy, 24 years old, with Erin and Jamie Richardson

Kimmy, 28 years old with Tammy, Mom, Suzanne, Kari, and Tiffany (puppy)

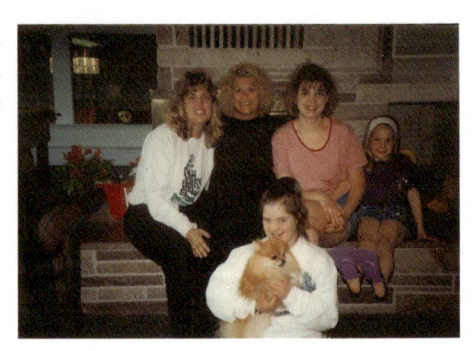

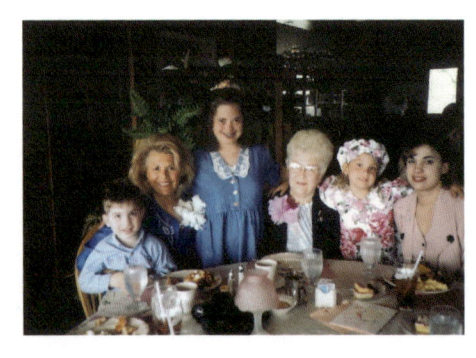

Mother Day 1996: Kimmy, 29 years old with Bret, Mom, Grandma Mathewson, Kari and Suzy.

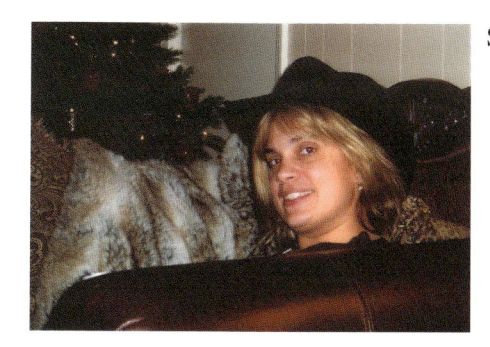

Sister Suzanne

Sister Suzanne with husband Dusty Miller

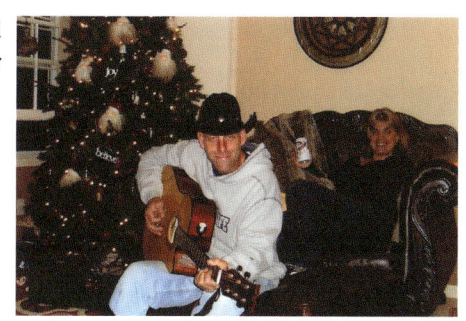

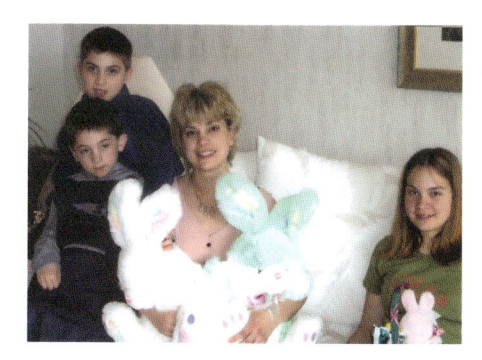

Sister Suzanne with her children Bret, Tyler, and Kari

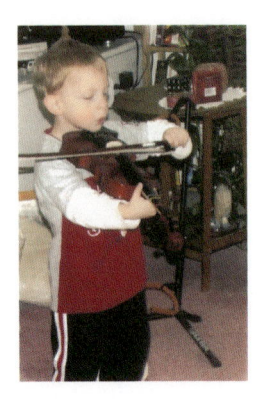

Brody, Kimmy's nephew
(Suzanne and Dusty's son)

Sister Tammy

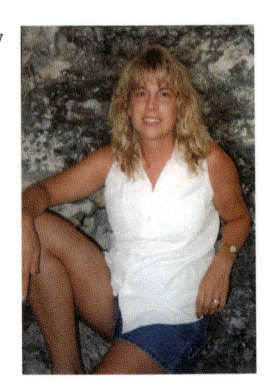

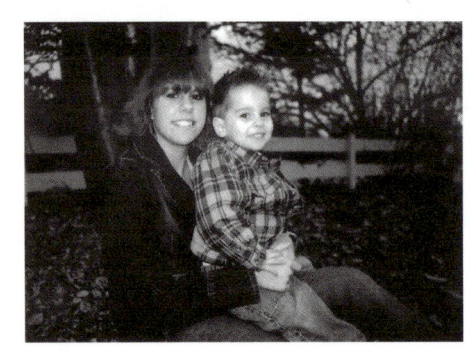

Tammy's daughter
Whitney and son Preston

Kimmy's Aunt Beverly
Mancuso with 2 of her
grandchildren

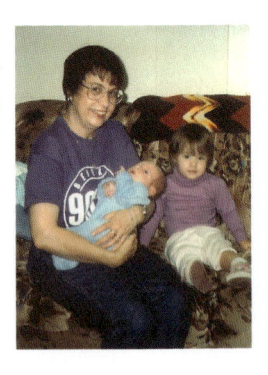

Judith E. Mathewson   35

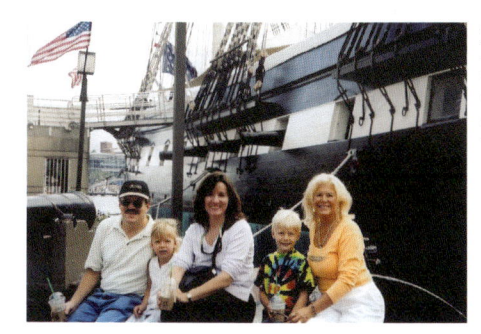

2003. Andrew, Allison, Maryann and Ryan Walker with Mom at Baltimore, Maryland.

Kimmy 36 years old with friends Ryan and Allison Walker, and Mom

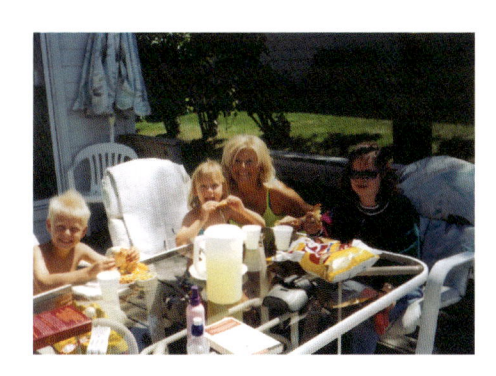

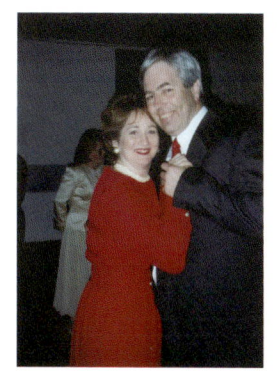

Mom's special friends, Tom and Jena Townsend

36   *Down Syndrome: Raising a Child Like Kimmy*

These pictures are only some of the special memories in Kimmy's life. My hope is that you will be blessed to see how normal her life is and how she is able to draw others into her life, just by being herself.

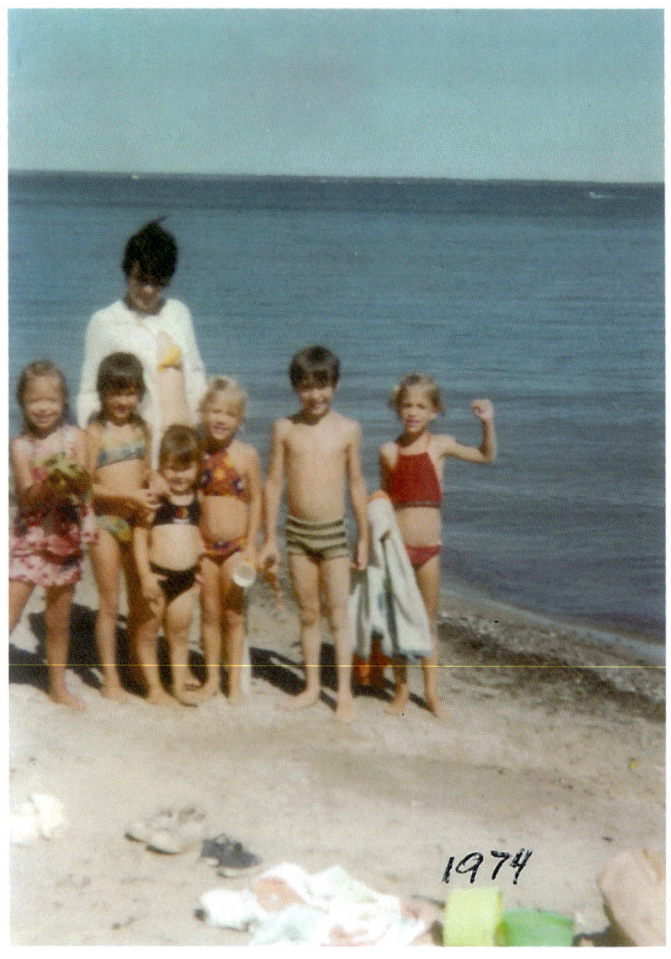

Kimmy, 7 years old, with Aunt Beverly Mancuso, Stacey, Kathy, Tammy, Todd and Suzy

Chapter 4

The Progressive Years

Everything Kimmy has accomplished has been major and a time to thank God for each miracle. Life was very difficult for her physically, as well as mentally, which made those accomplishments an event. Because Down syndrome so encircled her mind and body, no one knew what to expect of her capabilities until they sprung forth from her.

As a very young child, Kimmy had pointed at most of the things she wanted. She made a breakthrough when she could speak in a one-word sentence such as, bottle, water, soup, cake, up, down, etc. At three and a half, Kimmy spoke her first true grouping of words at Grandma and Grandpa Mathewson's house. She was beginning to crawl up the carpeted staircase by herself when I heard her say, "Mommy, want to go upstairs!" My mother and I looked at each other with tears in our eyes and smiled. We ran to Kimmy and I scooped her up in my arms, hugging and kissing her.

Kimmy was a sickly child and there were more times than not that I would lay her down to sleep by the side of my bed so I could hear if she was breathing okay. Sometimes, I needed to keep an eye on her or change her clothes and clean her up if vomiting occurred.

When she learned to talk, Kimmy began the next journey in her life—school. To start school, children had to be potty trained, which Kimmy was. Children also had to be able to communicate their needs by talking and walking, if a child could. And walk she did! Kimmy loved being mobile. She loved to ride her trike and get around without being carried or put into her baby walker.

By age seven, she was enrolled in the Pied Piper School and attended five days a week. She loved the bus ride, her school, her friends, and the gifted teachers. These caring, talented teachers were able to reach these children with such a wide span of mental and physical disabilities. Through their help over the years, Kimmy excelled in reading, writing, and social skills. Reading comprehension was not a strong point, but she would read and read. She would print various words, sentences, and paragraphs from books and the Bible onto paper. She wrote in run-on sentences without periods or paragraphs. Just words running into one another, but there was an interaction of thought patterns. She was content learning and was happy—isn't that what matters the most? Kimmy spent hours drawing lines down sheets of yellow legal paper. Once that was accomplished, she would fill in each space with a different colored crayon. Suzanne wanted to keep a memory of this daily activity, so Kimmy's teacher had some of these sheets laminated for table placemats for her children. She also made two for us that we still use today. As you can imagine, they are as colorful as a day filled with sunshine.

The years Kimmy attended the Pied Piper School were her active years. Between the ages of seven and eighteen, Kimmy had the joy and opportunity to be a cheerleader, play basketball, baseball, roller skate, and perform in school programs. The school also took the children on one-day school trips to visit various businesses and plants around town or to play in the parks on the swings and slides.

Kimmy enjoyed participating in many of the same activities that other children enjoyed. Each Sunday, she would choose one of her three Bibles to take with her to Sunday school. On Wednesday nights, she participated in Awana, a children's church activity. This was a night that the children, as well as the Awana teachers, looked forward to. The energy level was awesome and loud!

By far, her favorite church activity was being part of the annual Christmas program. Her participation ranged from being an angel to singing in the children's Christmas choir. This was a learning experience for the choir director as well. He learned not to put the microphone in front of her. She would sing with all her heart, but you could not understand a word she sang. But God knew, and He was always smiling down on her!

Another year, Kimmy was encased in a big box wrapped in bright red paper with a large gold bow tied on top of her head. With an ear-to-ear grin, she led the procession of children down the aisle to present these gifts to the Christ child who lay peacefully in the manger.

There were other times that Kimmy was able to let her light shine. She was selected to pose with a black Labrador puppy that was being auctioned during a Hospital Auxiliary Christmas

Tree Ball. She was just the right person to be selected to perform this task. Kimmy looked so pretty in her green velvet dress and carried the puppy with great pride and care (with my assistance) around to the various tables. People seemed more attracted to Kimmy than the little puppy that was auctioned and brought in more money than we had anticipated.

Tammy loved to teach Kimmy how to mime and make hand gestures. Once they did a song together called "Bull Frogs and Butterflies." It was incredibly cute seeing them put so much into their performance. Tammy spent a lot of her spare time playing with Kimmy. She also made sure that when her friends were at the house, Kimmy was included too. These are memories that remain imprinted in my mind and heart. From the time Kimmy was able to sit up, she loved the water. She has experienced the pleasures of a child's small outdoor plastic swimming pool, the large lakes that surround Michigan, and the various lakes within Michigan and other states. In my childhood, I was on a swim team and later became a life guard. I taught Kimmy how to swim, and she swam with ease, especially under water.

One time, my mom and sister, Beverly, took her three children and my three children to the lake for the afternoon while I was at work. Everyone was having fun until they noticed seven-year-old Kimmy was nowhere to be seen. My mom later said she died inside when they realized Kimmy was missing. Panic-stricken, my mother and sister called all the kids together. Beverly had a death grip on our mother's arm and was a basket case. She directed all of the kids to remain together as they walked the beach searching for Kimmy amongst the crowd of people in the water as well as those playing in the sand on the beach. They found Kimmy happily sitting in sand with another child and innocently building a sand castle. Mom and Beverly broke down and cried with relief at this scene.

Another traumatic scare occurred when Kimmy was three. Kimmy was dehydrated from vomiting and required more care and tests than the hospital was able to provide. The doctor called for an ambulance to take us to a larger hospital. During Kimmy's stay, an intern would come in periodically to check on her status. Three years later this same intern became her family physician in Alpena, Michigan. And she continued to be his patient for at total of thirty-three years.

The doctors at the second hospital began their various tests and x-rays. These tests revealed that through the many years that Kimmy pulled herself across our shag carpet at our home and the homes of family and friends, she had picked up and placed into her mouth not just the threads from the carpet, but also, coins, rubber bands, hair, and other small objects. The hospital staff explained that operating on her to remove the coins and other objects was not possible. Because of her heart condition, she would not survive the anesthesia, let alone the operation. They stated their hope that these items would attach to the lining of the stomach. However, if an item moved to the upper bowel track, it could block the entrance and could kill her. With this dismal projection, we continued with our day-to-day life praying that those objects would not move toward the bowel track opening. To this day, she has coins embedded in the lining of her stomach.

When Kimmy was sixteen, I received a call from school that Kimmy had passed out when she was roller skating in the gym. They had carried her up to a cot in one of the classrooms.

I picked up Kimmy from school and rushed her to the emergency room. Upon our arrival, the doctor on call contacted Kimmy's doctor and pediatric cardiologist to discuss this situation. They concluded that her body was not producing enough oxygen to sustain her activity level. Her breathing level capacity had dropped to 67, which was far too low to sustain her. This caused her to pass out. A normal, healthy person has an oxygen level of 96. While Kimmy had never achieved that breathing level, she breathed easily at around 86, but a level of 67 was too low. With the help of an oxygen concentrator that pumps oxygen into her body, Kimmy's breathes in oxygen at level of 83 to 86 to sustain her life. School became a non-issue since her body now required more rest. Three-hour naps became a part of Kimmy's life. She began at an oxygen concentrator level of 3. She is now at 6 or 7 depending on the blueness or coloration of skin and her social activity for any given day. A twenty-foot-long clear oxygen tube is attached from the concentrator to her nose through a nasal cannula. This provides her with the mobility to move about the house and gives her body the required level of oxygen. When Kimmy goes out of the house, she is switched to a portable oxygen unit. This allows her to go with me on errands and visit her Grandma Mathewson and other family and friends.

In 2002, my daughter Suzanne was staying with Kimmy for a couple of days. I was taking my second husband, Russ, across the state for a doctor's appointment regarding his health concerns. At 5:30 A.M. on Friday, Suzanne heard a loud thud on the floor above her bedroom. She entered Kimmy's bathroom and found her passed out in a pool of blood. She quickly called 911. They told her to take Kimmy to the hospital that was just a mile from our house. Suzanne quickly explained Kimmy's condition and the need for an ambulance to be dispatched to our home immediately.

Suzanne's next call was to me. I left my spouse to call a friend to borrow a vehicle to get him to his appointment. The drive home took me two hours. The thought of losing Kimmy and not being there when she needed me pulled at my conscience. Suzanne was in the process of taking a nursing course at the community college so I knew she could handle things until I made it to the hospital. When I did arrive, Kimmy had been put on an oxygen level of 12 and was incoherent and pale. I feared the worst.

Upon talking to the doctors, they were at a loss as to what was causing the bleeding. They also were in a dilemma as to how to determine what was causing it. The bleeding still had not stopped, but the flow had slowed down somewhat.

They consulted with her pediatric cardiologist to discuss what could be done without putting Kimmy under anesthesia. But anesthesia was the only option. It would be very risky and there was a high probability that she would not survive. She had so much going against her with two holes in her heart, lungs that were deteriorating, and the unknown cause for the bleeding.

The decision was made to put a scope down her throat and look for the possible cause of the bleeding. The next step was to pull a team of doctors together to perform the procedure. Surgeries were never scheduled on Saturdays. Therefore, calls were placed for doctors, nurses, and an anesthesiologist to be in place for Saturday morning. Another decision was made that

Kimmy would be placed under a very low dose of anesthesia that would put her in a light sleep state.

It was a long, agonizing night. Kimmy was still bleeding, unconscious, pale, and lifeless. As I stayed with her all night, I talked to her and held her hand. I tried to reassure her, as well as myself, that she would be fine. I begged her to just hold on. Most of the family was with me Saturday morning. We were all pulling for her, Grandma Mathewson, my sister, Suzanne and her children, and a brother-in-law and his wife. My husband, who was not good with scary situations like this would arrive later. For thirty-five years, I had taken care of Kimmy and I knew that Russ would be there when he felt comfortable with her situation. We'd been married for twenty-three years, and I knew his heart was there even though he was not. He had his own ways of caring and that is what mattered.

As for the rest of us, we sat in the waiting room for what seemed like hours, but only one hour had passed. We were filled with relief when we were informed the surgery was over. They had found and removed a corroded, razor-sharp penny that had sliced the lining. Fortunately, it would not need to be cauterized since the swelling of the bleeding area would allow for it to mend on its own. This was one of the coins Kimmy had swallowed some twenty years earlier while pulling herself across the floors of ours and others homes. The doctor stated that there were other coins and objects embedded in the lining of her stomach, but that there was no threat of them moving to cause her damage in the future. He added that they had kept talking to her while performing the scope. When they had removed the object. even though she was in a light sleep state, he had asked her if she wanted to see it. She had responded with a raspy "yes," then looked at the penny and said, "cool," before falling back to sleep.

After an hour in recovery, she was returned to her room. She was totally wiped out and groggy, but alive! As in the past, the doctors shook their heads in amazement, but I knew that God was the amazing one. He had used those doctors to bring Kimmy through yet another death-defying experience.

Additional blood tests were necessary to ensure that the function levels of her body were within their normal range. Those tests revealed that her hemoglobin level had dropped drastically enough to require two blood transfusions. Extra amounts of potassium also needed to be pumped back into her. After a few days, she was in stable condition and allowed to come home—if an oxygen equipment company could supply frozen liquid oxygen to our home. Kimmy now required a concentrated oxygen level supply of twelve in order to keep her in a stable condition. And the only way that could be provided was to find a source for frozen liquid oxygen. We accomplished this with the help of another company that had provided her with her past oxygen needs.

The oxygen company arrived at our house. After much conversation, they decided the best way to get the long hoses into the house and to Kimmy's bedroom (without having to set the three frozen containers inside the house) was to drill a hole large enough to bring for the hose through the window frame. After pulling the hoses through this hole, and setting up the other necessities they left to bring Kimmy home from the hospital. With the setup of the new equipment complete, these professional staff employees from the oxygen company explained how this new process of oxygen was going to work.

In approximately three days, the three tanks would be empty and I would need to switch to three new tanks. That meant the twelve large tanks that were placed under our car port area would be empty in three days. They would come back on that third day and bring another supply of twelve tanks. This process continued for three months until her oxygen level consumption was back to level 5 again.

Kimmy required care for twenty-four/seven for the next three months. Slowly, week by week, she began the recovery process. She was so weak and white, so frail and exhausted that only time would tell if she would have any after effects and what it meant in terms of her life expectancy.

Initially, I used baby monitors so I could always be assured of hearing her movements or whispers. Eventually, she was able to ring a little hand bell to get my attention. She went from a bed pan to the potty chair to a wheel chair to make it to the bathroom. I spoon fed her soft foods and gradually worked up to more solid foods.

Home health care providers made periodic checks on her vital signs and exercised her legs and arms because the muscles were weak from not being used. And by doing these exercises, her body would be ready as her condition improved.

After six months, Kimmy was almost as healthy as she was before this ordeal. Her oxygen intake had returned to a level 5. Eating everyday food became normal again, and her alertness and color was back. Her social activity was minimized. Keeping her in a more consistent low profile for awhile longer was best for her health and well-being. Within a year, she was back to her previous health status. Once again, God had His hand upon her and gave her the determination to live despite another setback. There was a need to increase Kimmy's medications in order to help her organs to function at their optimum level. She was put on a daily intake of seventeen pills. To this day, her intake remains the same unless, of course, her body is retaining too much fluid or she has developed a cold or such. Then more medications or shots are required. Thank God for the wisdom He gave to doctors to be able to monitor a person's bodily functions by taking simple blood tests.

During this time, I loved God and talked to Him, but I did not have a personal relationship with Him until thirteen years after Kimmy was born. It was at this time that I accepted Christ as my personal Savior and into my heart.

Remembering that monumental day is like it happened yesterday, but it was on January 28, 1980. At a Sunday morning service, the pastor gave the altar call and God came into

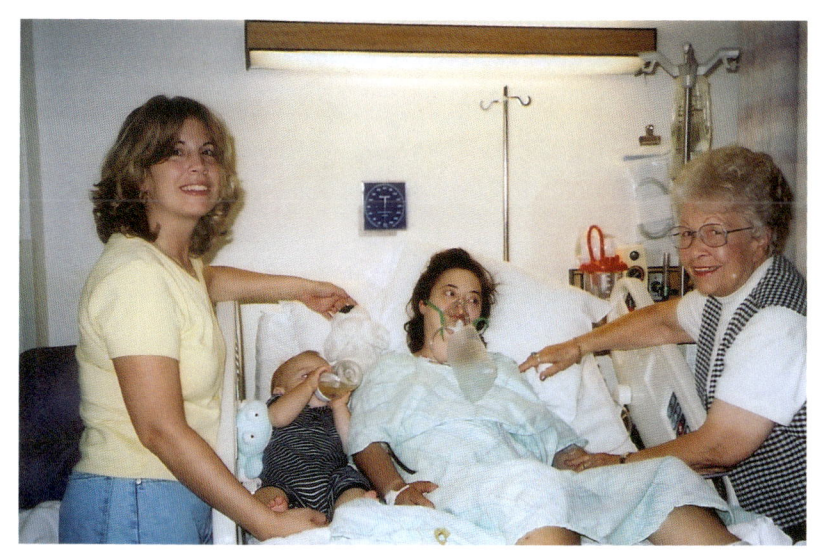

Kimmy, 35 years old, with sister Tanmy, nephew Preston, and Grandma Mathewson

my heart. I can remember a couple of deacons taking me into a room off from the altar. They asked me what my favorite scripture was and I answered, "What's a scripture?" I came to God as a lost sheep and He took me into His loving arms.

Six months later, my children, my husband, and I walked into Lake Huron to be water baptized. He still has His arms wrapped around me, guiding, nudging, and nurturing my spiritual growth. God knows our needs even when we do not know Him. He answers prayers and is beside us all the time. He is waiting for each of us to accept Him as our personal savior. No matter what our situation, He will never leave or forsake us.

Chapter 5

Personality Plus

Over the years, Kimmy's heart condition worsened due to the fact that her heart had to pump hard to get the blood flow past the two holes. Thus, the heart worked overtime. This made her life expectancy even more of an uncertainty. Scar tissue had already built up, and it continues to build up in the arteries. When the heart pumps the blood as hard as it can into the arteries, the artery entrances become smaller as the scar tissue increases. In turn, this causes a lack of oxygen that was already at a low level before.

This lack of oxygen is the culprit that causes the blueness in Kimmy's lips and fingers, the dark circles around her eyes, and causes her to be more lethargic. Some days are worse than others. But on her good days, Kimmy looks as pink and pretty as a newborn baby.

When the blueness appears, her activity level slows down. This is the lethargic part caused by the lack of oxygen throughout her body. The body does this naturally. Keeping Kimmy in a calming atmosphere has helped. This slows down the hard pumping action of her heart, which deprives her of the oxygen that she so desperately needs to survive.

Kimmy can be easily upset and her feelings hurt. Trying to raise her without being overly protective has been a challenge. Having given birth to three children in twenty-six months, I tried, as much as possible, to raise them with the same guidelines, love, and care.

This would have been difficult in normal living conditions. Add to that, ten years of abuse. Trying to keep a calm atmosphere for the children became almost impossible. To protect the children, I became more of a passive individual thinking the abuse would lessen. Did this help? Somewhat, but the children cannot remember any of their years before the age of seven. And, that was my youngest child's age when I filed for divorce.

Still, it was important to keep the guidelines of acceptable behavior the same for all. Praise, words of encouragement, and nap and bed times were the same for my three girls. I wanted to be sure that no one felt unloved or felt there was any favoritism toward Kimmy. Which, as I think back, was never the case, for we all helped one another. Suzy and Tammy were a breath of life for Kimmy. They would spend their time playing, singing, and laughing. We enjoyed all the simple things that normal families do together. And we never gave it a thought that our day-to-day life was any different than that of other families. This was our natural way of life, and we enjoyed that life together.

Suzanne and Tammy were, and still are positive, fun loving, and totally caring of their sister Kimmy. The time they are able to spend together has always been uplifting to Kimmy emotionally, physically, and spiritually. She loves the interaction. Sometimes she rides behind Tammy on the four-wheeler with an oxygen tank tucked between Tammy's leg and the frame of the four-wheeler. Going somewhere special with Sue brings an ear-to-ear grin and a twinkle to her eye.

In Kimmy's opinion, food would be number one on her list of things she likes best. Kimmy is always alert enough to catch the words "time to eat" or "let's go out to eat." Her favorite foods are Mexican taco salad or fajitas. Chinese food, usually a combination of shrimp and noodles, comes in second. Italian food with shrimp, is in third on her list.

There were times, I'd swear, that Kimmy would look down the price column first and select the most expensive item on the menu. My reaction, of course, was to say, "I think it best I help you choose." Then I'd give her the choice of three entrées from the menu. She'd give me a hurt look, with her eyes cast down, but would finally decide on one of the items I'd selected. I would hide the chuckle that was rising within me, knowing we would go through this same procedure the next time we'd go out to eat.

It is amazing that even after this many years, she has never faltered very much from her past thinking or pattern of living. But, there are those moments of surprise. There were moments when Kimmy showed a change in attitude and her little stubborn streak would come out. This is what I considered the teenager inside her. She would roll her eyes or march stiffly down the hallway to her bedroom. If she didn't like what I offered her for lunch, she was not shy about saying, "I'm not hungry!" This was her way of letting me know that she had something else in mind for lunch. Sometimes, she set the food out on the counter as her way of telling me what she wanted to eat. Usually, I tried to give Kimmy a couple of choices, but there were times when this was not possible. When I could not, she would eventually give in and eat what was placed in front of her. These days are few and far between, but they do happen. I try to find the right way to handle it and get her through that current situation without frustration on either of our parts.

Recently, I was in the kitchen. Out of the corner of my eye, I saw an object flying across the hallway into my bedroom. Kimmy was standing in her bedroom doorway with a frustrated look on her face. When she gets this way, I talk calmly to her until she soothes down and can let me know what has upset her. This time, the object was her watch. She was upset that it was not working. I gently explained that the battery needed to be replaced, and I would get a new battery to put in it. Knowing how important the watch was to Kimmy, I replaced the battery that day.

Kimmy was so relieved. She smiled and cried as she flung her arms around my waist. Kimmy runs her life (and mine) by that watch. She knows that 7:00 A.M. is the time for her to get up and lunch time is 12:00 P.M. When it is 1:00 P.M., it is nap time, and 3:30–4:00 P.M. is time to get up from her nap and have a snack. Dinner is at 5:30–6:00 P.M. After dinner she gets into her pajamas. At 7:30 P.M., she can have a can of soda; at 8:15 P.M., she can have a cup of ice cream or sugar free gelatin. At 8:30 P.M., she walks down the hall to begin her ritual of getting ready for bed.

Kimmy's nightly process consists of pulling her bedspread down and spending the other twenty-five minutes on the potty, talking, singing, or just thinking. When this is complete, she calls out to me, "I'm ready!"

That is my cue to walk down the hall. Smiling, I enter her room and take her little socks off—at the age of 41, Kimmy's feet are still a child's size 3. The next part of the ritual is to remove her watch, bring the covers up to her chin, snuggle her down, and say prayers with her. We ask for God's protective hedge to be placed around her and our house and His healing hand upon her body. We pray for her sisters and their children. We ask for His guidance in our lives. We always remember to ask God to give Grandma Mathewson a big hug from us and to let her know that she is loved and missed. After turning out the light, I kiss Kimmy on the cheek telling her that I love her. When she replies that she loves me, I tease her by saying, "I love you more!" With this, she giggles, finds my fingers, and squeezes them with her little hand.

These times are always special to me. They are memories that I can hold onto at any moment and feel the love flow through my body, making life worth living. Everyday, God has given us is a gift. Whatever days He has left for us, we will treasure.

Chapter 6

Southern Living

In 2006 my husband and I filed for a mutually agreed upon separation and divorce. This same year Kimmy and I moved to South Carolina to live near my third daughter, Tammy. In doing so this helped to keep familiarity and consistency in Kimmy's life. Then in 2007, my second daughter, Suzanne moved to Florida. We have enjoyed being able to visit and tour around the various areas of the southeastern part of the states. The warmer weather agrees with Kimmy's health condition. The cold weather had made it difficult, at times, for her to go outside. It is better for Kimmy to be in a warmer climate were she can be more mobile. This also makes it easier on her deteriorating lungs and overworked heart.

The move to the south naturally brought on the search for a new church. A priority was to find a church where Kimmy would be accepted, treated well, and taught with love and care. There were many wonderful churches, but I chose the Alice Drive Baptist Church.

They offer a fantastic Awana children's program. More

importantly, the leader and children are very accepting of Kimmy. In particular, one little African-American girl pushes Kimmy around in her wheelchair to ensure Kimmy is involved in the less physical activities. They all have a wonderful time playing games, earning play money to shop at their Awana Store, and learning about God's word. Miss Pat, Kimmy's Sunday School teacher, possesses a loving, caring, and serving nature. She has a true heart for Kimmy, who returns that love.

The way in which Pastor Clay presents God's word and his teachings continue to challenge and guide me through everyday life. This also keeps me connected to God's principles. The church offers a Sunday Single's Bible Study and a Tuesday evening gathering called Oasis. Other social gatherings keep a member's life filled all year.

At one of the Tuesday night singles meetings, I met, "Ba," who became my closest friend. She is Vietnamese, and a beautiful person inside and out. Ba, her parents, sisters, and brothers have taken Kimmy and me into their lives as though we were family. An exceptional individual, Ba always thinks of and puts others before herself—selflessly and with love. We have spent birthdays, Christmas Eve, and Easter Day together. Kimmy is loved and accepted by all the children. Each year, Ba has made sure that an area of the Easter egg hunt has been created just for Kimmy. The nieces and nephews know this is special treatment, but they accept this because of their compassion for Kimmy and the enjoyment in watching her participate with them.

I have made a Kimmy scrapbook that holds the special things she has done or made. I have also included some special pictures and cards that I cherish. The scrapbook would not be

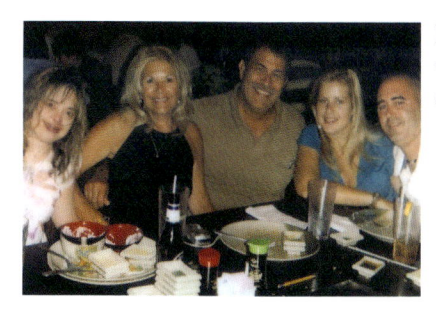

Kimmy's "41st" birthday dinner with Mom, Tony Alicia, Rachel and Michael Swansona

Kimmy's 41st birthday party

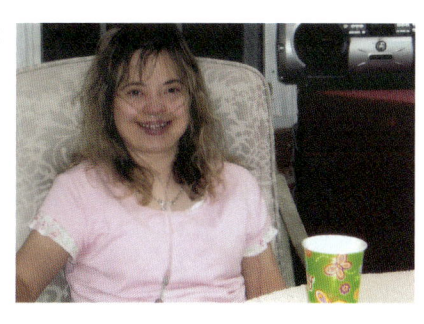

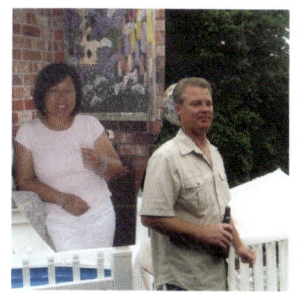

Kimmy's 41st birthday party with BA and Wayne

Kimmy's 41st birthday party with David and Kathi

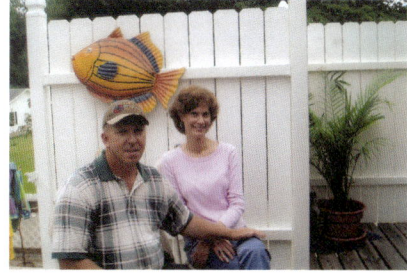

complete without the penny (in a plastic baggie) that was pulled out of her upper bowel track in 1992. That penny caused so much bleeding and almost took her life. Many other memories fill the pages of the book that bulges at its seams. Hopefully, there will be many more memories to include on the empty pages.

This scrapbook will be passed down to Suzanne and Tamara as a reminder of how special their sister Kimmy was and what an impact she had upon their lives. The scrapbook can be shared with their children and grandchildren. Kimmy is a breath of life from God. He intended for her to be shared until that time He takes her home to the Kingdom of Heaven forever.

Kimmy is my precious gift of life from God.

The following pictures are just a few memories from Kimmy's scrapbook.

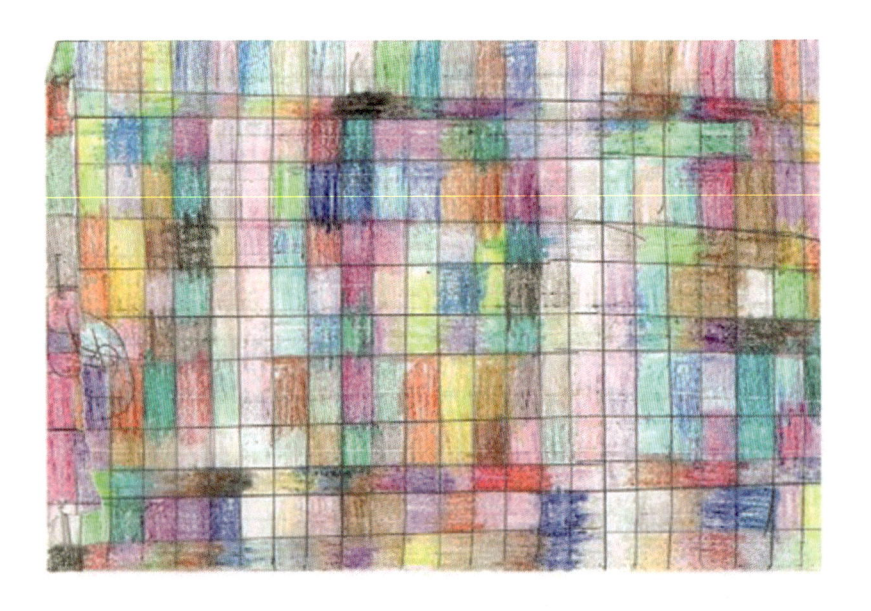

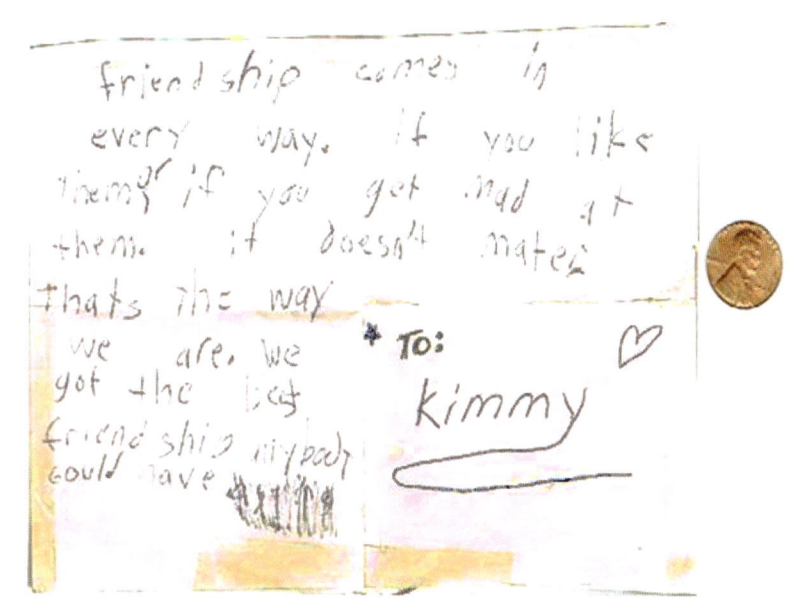

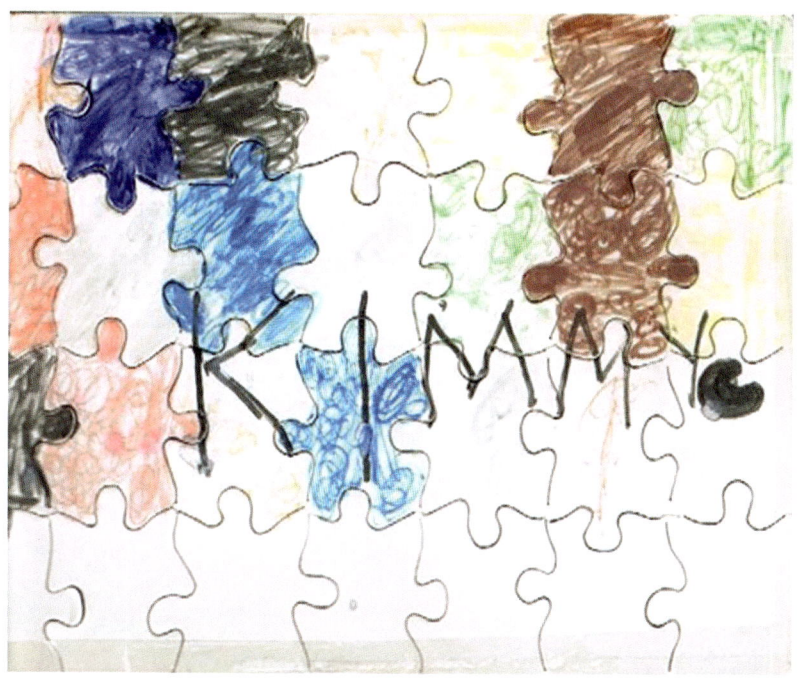

friendship comes in every way. if you like them, if you get mad at them. it doesn't mater thats the way we are, we got the best friendship anybody could have

TO: kimmy

Some of Kimmy's Bible W[ork]

GOD'S WORD — — THE BIBLE

TAKE-TIME

1. TO PRAY GOD REQUIRES IT
2. TO READ THE BIBLE IT'S GOD'S WO[RD]
3. TO GO TO CHURCH WE NEED
4. THE FELLOWSHIP TO MAKE GO[D]
5. FREINDS IT MAKES II FE WOR[K]
6. LIVING TO RES[T] OUR BODY REQUI[RES]
7. TO SMILE IT BRIGHTENS TH[E]
8. LIVES OF OTHERS TO TELL
9. YOU FAMILY MEMBERS
10. YOU LOVE THEM TO ENJO[Y]
11. NATURE IT'S GOD'S GIFT TO YOU
12. TO BE KIND TO YOUR PETS
13. IT WARMS THEIR HEARTS
14. TO FEED THE BIRDS GOD HA[S]
15. THIS DEEP TO BLOW THE DU[ST]
16. OFF YOUR MIND READ GOOD
17. BOOKS TO VIST THE A[GED]
18. SOME WILL BE TOO OLD
19. TO HELP THE BEREAVED WE
20. SHALL BE THERE TO ENJO[Y]
21. TO @ THE SICK OUR
22. DAILY WILL

You May Say

by Judith Mathewson,
proud mother of Kimberly

You may say, "Why me?"
You may think why has this happen, what have I done?
Not knowing this is God's Plan.
You may say, "I can't do this!"
You may think this is much too hard!
Not knowing God has His hand on you
And you are part of His Plan.
You may say, "But, why has He chosen me?"
You may think someone else is better qualified.
Not knowing God's saying "you" are His Plan.
You may say, "But I have nothing to give."
You may think What is God thinking?!
But God is saying,
"This is my blessing that I have bestowed upon you!
"This is my gift,
This precious buddle that will count on your love
And your care for life itself.
"This is my Plan,
And you are the chosen one to walk this walk,
Because you are love exemplified
Through this 'Little Angel'
"And all who come in contact
With her will be touched.
Touched, by the hand of God.
"This, this is My Plan,
My Plan for your life."

Chapter 7

Expectations—Have None!

How would I respond if someone asked me what they needed to do or know in raising a special needs child? I could only make suggestions that stem from my own recollections and decisions on how I sustained and raised Kimmy. Forty-one years ago, there were no books on "How To" or "What To Expect, From Your Special Needs Child." For me, survival and a mother's natural intuition came into play in the raising of Kimmy.

I can emphasize the importance of finding a sensitive, caring, and knowledgeable cardiologist and family physician. Those doctors will know what tests need to be done and the hospital that can best perform them. There will be blood work, x-rays, electrocardiograms (EKGs), echocardiogram (echogram), oxygen level findings, etc. It is anguishing to watch your child go through so much. It is difficult to calm the tears and fears of another when you are at your own breaking point. That is something I would not wish on anyone. But as a parent, you do it for your unaware and fearful child. Comfort, love, and a soft reassuring voice can greatly help your child past these endless days of testing.

When all the results are available, the doctors will review your child's case, tell you what, if any, heart condition there may be. You will learn if there is a lung deficiency or if any of the child's vital organs are not functioning properly. At some point, you may be given a heart-wrenching prognosis on your child's life expectancy, which can only be offered with uncertainty.

When you leave the hospital, you know your child's future is unforeseeable. But right now, you have a basic understanding of your child's physical condition and a handful of prescriptions to help maintain and keep your child's body functioning in, as much as possible, a balanced condition.

No physician can determine or judge what your child's mental capability will be. As your child ages and tries various challenges, a prognosis may be given of the age level that may be attained. So you encourage, guide, and see that your child receives physical therapy when it is needed. It is also important to learn the recommended weight for your child and, to the best of your ability, keep to the weight that the doctor recommends. This may vary depending upon heart and lung issues.

Although Kimmy is forty-one years old, she physically looks to be twelve years old. Mentally, she varies between the ages of four and eight. This is dependent upon the mental challenges at hand or the mental capability within the different situation or activity she is involved in at that moment. People are always surprised to learn that she is forty-one years old and often give her a double or triple look! Her weight stays around

106 pounds. This is the optimum weight she should carry for her heart and lung conditions. It is also important to raise a special needs child in the same way you would a "normal" child. This helps in obtaining a maximum mental and physical growth. It also helps them in preparation for school, social activities, and social functions, such as going to restaurants, friends' or families' homes, various parties, church, etc.

If you have other children, you want them to feel you are not "playing favorites." This could and does happen if their rules are different than those you have for your special needs child. Your other children need to feel loved and that you are just as excited and thrilled over their accomplishments. Also, being consistent with unacceptable behavior is important. What is most important is to raise your special needs child as you would a normal child, keeping their health condition as a continuous guideline.

As in most families, parents have their disagreements and conflicts. It is a fact of life and needs to be addressed. Keep arguments from the ears and eyes of your disabled children who tend to be emotional and highly sensitive to anger through loud voices and/or physical attacks. They feel a sense of fear. Depending on the degree or level of a child's Down syndrome, anxiety can be detrimental to their health. I know this from my own experience in an abusive marriage.

In my opinion, any physiologist or doctor would recommend that arguments of any degree should be kept not only from your normal healthy children, but especially from a complex, sensitive disabled child. What your child does need is consistency, stability, fulfillment, encouragement, and a lot of love.

Many Down syndrome children have no concept of time as in hours, days, weeks, etc.. Their time frame is gauged within their own body. But they may have an uncanny ability to anticipate an event, a meal out, an arrival of a package, and holidays—especially birthdays and Christmas, since these two represent presents to them!

I have found that relating an event to Kimmy no more than two days (sometimes, two hours) before is best for her level of anticipation. Letting her know any sooner would only let her down emotionally. Sometimes, I would slip and tell her in the morning what we were doing that evening. Then, as usual, I would help her get dressed for the day before getting dressed myself. Invariably, I would walk out of my bedroom and find her sitting at the kitchen counter waiting to go with her coat and shoes on. How sad she looked when I had to tell her we were not going yet, and she needed to take her coat and shoes off. I would reassure her that when it was time to leave that evening, she could put them back on.

By holding off on telling her about the upcoming events I have accomplished two things. First, I have given her something to anticipate or look forward to that day. More importantly, it gives her time to enjoy the anticipation, within a short timeframe that she can happily manage. Doing those two things eliminates Kimmy's emotional stress and disappointment level. And remember, everyone likes to be surprised whether or not they are disabled. We like the unexpected—whether it be gifts or events.

Try to get your child out of the house three or four times a week. This may mean doing errands with you, going to a playground, going shopping, or any small adventure like picking up fall leaves from your yard. Any of these could be a high point of their day. Think about it, how you would feel if all you saw was the inside of your home? Their life needs are similar to our own. They need the same distractions and feeling of mobility as we do. It is just that they have to depend on us to make these things possible for them. They might not be able to express their needs as we do, nor can they get out and about without our assistance, but those needs are there. We need to remember that we are their arms and legs. We need to be conscious of this so we can help them to feel a fulfillment in their own life.

Another very important subject is the ability to trust. Kimmy trusts me explicitly. I remember telling my friends, "Kimmy has such a trust in me that I could tell her to stand in the middle of the street. Not only would she would do it, but she would stay there until I told her to come back to me." I never would have done that, but it explains the level of trust she has in me. Therefore, I need to make sure that all my promises are kept. She needs to know that when she is sick, I will be by her side and continuously take care of her. Whether she is depressed, scared, or unknowing of what is happening around her, she knows she can depend on my love. I will always be there for her.

There are various levels of Down syndrome, so it is very important to have "no expectations" when it pertains to their mental or physical capabilities. Allow each advancement that they make in life to be a milestone. For it is, especially to them. It is their milestone, and it is your overwhelming happiness for them that lets them feel more of the joy over their recent accomplishment.

Sometimes these achievements come slowly, possibly six or eight months between each achievement—or more. But do not become discouraged. They may or may not advance to the degree you expect them to for their age. Just love and encourage them; play games and laugh together; give them all the hope you can muster up. Be there for them, be their cheerleader. But, have no expectations. Life is short. Enjoy and embrace your special needs child with all the caring, giving, and love that God has bestowed upon you. He chose you above all other people to care for this child. That alone will sustain you in the hours, days, weeks, months, and years to come.

Kimmy is my blessing, and I hope you will be blessed by the writings within this small book. These memories bring forth both tears and joy for me, but mostly joy! As I was going through some books and writing, a piece of folded paper fell out of one of the books. Upon opening it up, tears came to my eyes. I know now, without a doubt, that God has had his hand upon my life and that He had chosen me to raise Kimmy, my own special little angel.

In closing, may God's hand be upon your life as it has been upon mine and Kimmy's. God bless and keep you in His loving hands. My love goes out to all parents of a special needs child. Please accept this special poem as my gift to you. With all my love, Judy

Special Parents For Sam

by Judith Mathewson

*There are memories to cherish,
To be shared or carried.
Words that are meant strictly
For encouragement.
Words about God's special plan
For a few special moms and dads.
For God has a child called Sam,
Who needs the tender care of
Parents somewhere.
So He says to an angel, "I'll give
Sam to Ann and Joseph over there.
"Since they have been given an
Abundance of love to share.
So, I'll give them this special
Child named Sam.
"For he will be perfect for
These exceptional parents,
Whom I have given the ability
To love and care for him
unconditionally.
"For not only will Sam be loved
In a moment,
But, he will be their joy,
Throughout every moment of their day.
"And they will tell others of
Their special son, so that whoever listens
Will trust in God's plan,
For they too may be given a special child
Like Sam!"*

The two appendices include forms that I have written up for use when I have had to be out of town. You may use these as a guideline for your own Special Needs Child.

Hopefully, these two forms will help give you guidance in the preparation when family members or qualified home health care service persons are needed.

Appendix I

EMERGENCY INFORMATION RECORD & AUTHORIZATION FOR EMERGENCY TREATMENT

Parent/Guardian Name: _____
Address: _____

Cell Phone: _____
Physician & Phone #: _____

Pediatric Cardiologist & Phone #: _____

Insurance Company & ID #: _____

Medicare A & D & ID #: _____

Dates I will be out of town: _____
Where I can be reached: _____
and on my cell: _____
Child's Name _____
Age _____ Birth Date _____
Allergies _____

Existing Medical Problems _____

Name of adult that may sign for emergency treatment in my absence:

Address _____

Phone # _____

Signature of parent/Guardian: _____

Date: _____

Judith E. Mathewson
Child Name: Kimberly _____

Appendix II

PERSONAL CARE INSTRUCTIONS

Social Security #: _____
Health Insurance: Medicare & Medicaid
Parent Name & Address: _____

ITEM	TIME	INSTRUCTIONS (Sample of Kimmy's)
Food	Breakfast 7:30 or 8:00	Stay with Kimmy when she eats. Breakfast consists of juice, cereal or canned Fruit or apple sauce. At every meal let her know just to eat as much as she is hungry for—which usually is not a lot.
Pills	Breakfast	2 Vitamins before she eats. 4 smaller pills after Breakfast. 2 larger pills after she washes up and dresses. Pills located in Morning Pill Box.
Clothing	Morning	Give her the choice between 2 tops. Jeans or Bibs, socks to wear. No shoes unless you take her out for lunch or a movie.
Food	Lunch 12:00 or 12:30	Again, stay with her. Lunch consists of soup & crackers or hot dog & chips or Lil' o & crackers with a small glass of milk or juice.
Nap	1:00–3:30 or 4:00	She likes to be tucked in and sleeps with one of her stuffed animals. Usually: JC (a pony)
Pills	After Nap	5 Pills—located in Afternoon Pill Box.
Snack	3:30 or 4:00	Her snack is a couple of cookies or jell-o cup. She usually will want water or juice at that time.
Dinner	Any Time between 5:30 & 6:30	Kimmy eats anything, so whatever you decide to cook for dinner will be fine. After dinner she gets her pj's on (she will ask you which ones to wear).
Evening Snack	7:00–8:00	pop, ice cream or jell-o.

Bed Time 8:30   Bedtime Pills located in Pill Box. Have her go to
& Pills   the bathroom, when sitting on bed take her socks off & put foot lotion on. Tuck her in & say a prayer for her.

Foods to AVOID: Nuts
Ice (crushed or cubes—absolutely NO ice). She has choked on ice several times.
Tough Meats
Pop Corn
String Beans

Limited Foods: Fatty Foods
Limit Sugar Foods (she may have a bowl of ice cream with topping or a couple cookies in the evening—if she wants—she may not want anything—but you can go ahead and have what you want yourself.
Deep Fried Foods (Instead Bake the French Fries in the Oven for instance.
Limit Milk to Cereal and 1 Glass at Lunchtime.
Limit Cheese intake (Pizza is ok, or Parma. on Spaghetti is fine).

Showers: Tuesday mornings and Friday mornings. Wash her hair and use a conditioner. Wash her body with the PhisoHex, this helps stop the spots from becoming a problem. You can then have her wash her face and hands herself. Kimmy will need assistance getting into the shower and out of the shower. She also needs you to dry her off, that is difficult for herto do herself. After she brushes her teeth and dresses, comb and

Comments: Stay with her when she eats and takes her medicine. She has occasionally thrown-up, and will need your assistance in cleaning herself up whatever area around her needs to be cleaned up.

Stomach Pains: Give her 1 Aspirin or a Minstrel Pill.

Doctor: Dr. Grunsky—Colonial Family Practice, 325 Broad St, Sumter; Phone: 803-773-5227

Doctor: Dr. Schuler—Pediatric Cardiologist @ Med. Bldg 1, Richland Hospital, Columbia, SC; Phone: 803-434-7991

Reliable Medical Equipment: Oxygen Concentrator—418 Broad St, Sumter; Phone: 803-934-9212

Immediate Help Please Contact The Following Individuals:

    Name   Address   Phone Number

1. _____
2. _____
3. _____